NOT ONLY A CURE

One may sum up the entire philosophy of acupuncture and Chinese healing by recalling the ancient Mandarins who paid their physicians to keep them in good health. When they fell into illness, they immediately stopped all payment.

Acupuncture is, above all, preventive medicine, and the patient is treated as a whole—body, mind, and spirit inseparable. There is a precept which applies to acupuncture as well as to all Chinese healing; the acupuncturist will admonish, "Curing is not so good as preventing, and preventing is not so good as taking care of oneself."

—Lucille Leong

Other SIGNET and MENTOR Books
You'll Want to Read

ACUPUNCTURE

A Layman's View

LUCILLE ANN LEONG

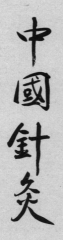

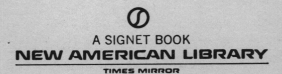

A SIGNET BOOK

NEW AMERICAN LIBRARY

TIMES MIRROR

DEDICATION

I dedicate this book to my mother, Rosa Leong. By her patience and love she has made this and much more possible.

It is fitting that the qualities of the best acupuncturist—perseverance, kindness, and a genuine love of mankind—should be her qualities too.

I take this opportunity to thank my mother for every inspiration she has given me.

 SIGNET TRADEMARK REG. U.S. PAT. OFF. AND FOREIGN COUNTRIES
REGISTERED TRADEMARK—MARCA REGISTRADA
HECHO EN CHICAGO, U.S.A.

SIGNET, SIGNET CLASSICS, SIGNETTE, MENTOR
and PLUME BOOKS are published by
The New American Library, Inc.
1301 Avenue of the Americas, New York, New York 10019

First Printing, February, 1974

3 4 5 6 7 8 9

PRINTED IN THE UNITED STATES OF AMERICA

CONTENTS

List of Illustrations vii

Foreword by Dr. Andrew Ming ix

Introduction xi

Chapter One
The West Gets the Point 15

Chapter Two
The Philosophy of Acupuncture
Yang and Yin 17
Ch'i and the Meridians 20
The Five Elements and Their Cycles 49

Chapter Three
Acupuncture in Practice
The Point 52
Needling 56
An Na and *Ai* 64
Diagnosis—the True Art 66
The Practitioner Himself 70

Chapter Four
From the Stone Age Onward 72

Chapter Five
Safe, Simple, Economical—Acupuncture
Anesthesia 75

Chapter Six
The Oriental Science in the Occident 80

Chapter Seven
Why Does It Work? 82

Chapter Eight
  What Acupuncture Can Cure:
    The Physiological Illness   87

Chapter Nine
  Not Magic   90

Chapter Ten
  The Future   98

Summary of Yang and Yin   118

Glossary   121

Bibliography   127

LIST OF ILLUSTRATIONS

FIGURE		PAGE
1.	Yin-Yang	18
2.	Yin-Yang and Trigrams	18
3.	The lung meridian, the large-intestine meridian	26–29
4.	The stomach meridian	30
5.	The spleen meridian	31–32
6.	The heart meridian	33
7.	The small-intestine meridian	34
8.	The bladder meridian	35
9.	The kidney meridian	36
10.	The pericardium (vascular system) meridian, the triple heater (hypothalamus) meridian	37
11.	The gallbladder meridian	38
12.	The liver meridian	39
13.	The governor-vessel meridian	40
14.	The conceptional-vessel meridian	41
15.	A view of the head with the meridians and acupuncture points	42
16.	A back view of the torso with the meridians and acupuncture points	43
17.	A front view of the torso with the meridians and acupuncture points	44
18.	A view of the arms with the meridians and acupuncture points	45
19.	A side view of the torso with the meridians and acupuncture points	46
20.	Inside and front views of the legs with the meridians and acupuncture points	47

FIGURE		PAGE
21.	Outside and back views of the legs with the meridians and acupuncture points	48
22.	The *sheng* and *k'o* cycles	50–51
23.	The *ts'un-fen* measurements and the meridians on the front of the body	54
24.	The *ts'un-fen* measurements and the meridians on the back and side of the body	55
25.	Gold needles and five- and seven-star needles	58
26.	Silver needles	58
27.	Stainless steel needles	59
28.	Very fine stainless steel needles	59
29.	Locating the point	60
30.	Inserting the needle	61
31.	Rotating the needle	62
32.	Rotating the needle	62
33.	Forty-five-degree angle of insertion	63
34.	Fifteen-degree angle of insertion	63
35.	*An na* instruments	65
36.	Burning *ai*	65
37.	Moxibustion	66
38.	A diagram of the pulses	68
39.	Chinese figurine with acupuncture meridians and points	92
40.	Chinese figurine with acupuncture meridians and points	93
41.	A life-size model with the acupuncture points	94
42.	A life-size model with the acupuncture points	95
43.	A life-size model with the acupuncture points (back view)	96
44.	A life-size model with the acupuncture points (side view)	97

FOREWORD
BY DR. ANDREW MING

I am very pleased and grateful that the American people are awakening to the value of the traditional healing art of acupuncture. At last, after thousands of years of success in China and widespread practice in foreign countries, American medical authorities are beginning to realize the benefits of acupuncture. Although acupuncture is a curative and preventive therapy, its greatest contribution to the West can be as a form of anesthesia. Acupuncture can accomplish these things by restoring balance to the body in compliance with the principles of natural laws. Therefore it is true when the Chinese say that acupuncture is the "science of sciences."

As an acupuncturist, I believe that this is a time for encouragement and caution. The very essence of acupuncture is its underlying philosophy and its love for humanity. In the rush and excitement of discovery, Americans must not enter into acupuncture without a full understanding of its essence. With much patience and receptivity, we can combine the art of acupuncture with Western medical science. This will be an unbeatable team with an unlimited future.

I have worked in depth with the author, Lucille, on this book; and I feel that she has perceived the real meaning of acupuncture from the practitioner's viewpoint. This book is a product of the knowledge and understanding which she has assimilated. It is an expression of her very nature: striving for excellence in learning and in character, a quality inseparable from a true acupuncturist.

This book is unique, since it is a view of acupuncture from the inside projected outward, instead of an outside view looking in. Most writings on acupuncture merely research and translate the Chinese texts; the best translation cannot grasp the full meaning. This book, since it is more than a translation, has the true understanding of the acupuncturist behind it.

It is my conviction that there is an Intelligence which is greater than man, an Intelligence which creates and heals. As an acupuncturist, I am but Its channel for healing. I consider myself blessed in being able to help people through the use of acupuncture.

DR. ANDREW MING
Chinese Traditional Medical
Doctor and Acupuncturist

傳統中醫師
蕪針灸主理
明明德

INTRODUCTION

Acupuncture has great promise for our modern medical world. Thousands of years have established it as a traditional healing in the Orient. Now a modern scientific approach can adapt it for the world's present and future medical needs. The West must neither ignore acupuncture nor rush recklessly into it. Certainly no one knows all the answers about acupuncture; but what we do know is that it works.

This book was written to dispel some of the myths and misapprehensions regarding acupuncture. The image of "human pincushions" which frightens some is an exaggeration arising from insufficient knowledge and understanding. Far from primitive needling, acupuncture is a sophisticated science-philosophy. All Western sciences originated as philosophy. The seventeenth-century scientists in Europe were called "natural philosophers." Since that time, however, most scientists have repudiated their philosophical source. Not so the Chinese —they retain the Taoist philosophy and its significance in all their sciences. Hence acupuncture is a science deeply rooted in philosophy.

The story behind this book is very interesting. It started as a senior project for the high school which I attended, Polytechnic School in Pasadena. A speech and this book (then in the form of a paper) brought so much interest and enthusiasm that I was encouraged to publish the writing. There are many whose attention and encouragement helped me: students, parents, school administrators, doctors, and others. The wise and gracious guidance of Dr. James C. Caillouette has been invaluable. For editing this book and for directing and inspiring me I owe him many thanks.

Above all, I wish to extend my gratitude to Dr. Andrew Ming and to his daughter, Charmmie Ming. Here are two generations of acupuncturists —the experienced master and his student. Dr. Andrew Ming is an acupuncturist of great skill and kindness. He happened to have been a student of my grandfather, Dr. Li T'ien Lu, at Shantung University in China before the Chinese Civil War. As a professor of chemistry and biology, Dr. Ming taught at several government and private colleges in Taiwan: Sheng-te Christian College, the National Defense College, and the Armed Forces Staff College. During twelve years of practice in the Acupuncture Hospital, Taipei, Taiwan, he conducted three acupuncture classes, teaching medical doctors and several European physicians. For his knowledge and experience he was appointed a commissioner of the Chinese Acupuncture Association in Taiwan. His daughter, Charmmie Ming, after more than ten years of training from her father, is an acupuncturist in her own right and a member of the Chinese Acupuncture Association. The traditional art of acupuncture has been in the Ming family for generations. My deepest thanks to these two people for all their patience and help.

By active cooperation, traditional acupuncturists and open-minded medical doctors can make acupuncture a wise and widespread course of healing. Thoughtful consideration, research, and experimentation will win acupuncture a respected status in the modern medical world. I hope that this book will open more minds to the promise of acupuncture.

LUCILLE ANN LEONG

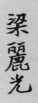

CHAPTER ONE

The West Gets the Point

"Getting the needle," [1] "a prickly panacea," [2] mysterious needles—all these epithets refer to the practice of acupuncture. American interest in acupuncture and the resulting rumors and half-truths have arisen fairly recently. The political recognition of Red China has led to a medical recognition. In May, 1971, at Peking, Dr. Arthur Galston of Yale and Dr. Ethan Singer of MIT witnessed the use of acupuncture as the sole anesthetic in the removal of a baseball-sized ovarian cyst.[3] In the same year, four American medical men—Drs. Samuel Rosen, Paul Dudley White, E. Grey Dimond, and Victor Sidel—viewed various major operations in-

[1] Michael Cusack, "Acupuncture—Is Getting the Needle Good for You?", *Science World*, XXIV (May 15, 1972), 9.
[2] "A Prickly Panacea Called Acupuncture," *Life*, LXXI (August 13, 1972), 32.
[3] "The Chinese Surgeons," *Newsweek*, LXXVII (June 7, 1971), 78.

volving acupuncture anesthesia. The ancient art of healing was further popularized by *New York Times* reporter James Reston. Recovering from an emergency operation for appendicitis in Peking, he was relieved of postoperative pain by an acupuncture treatment. Three needles were inserted into his right elbow and into an area below the knee. When twisted to "stimulate the intestine," they sent "ripples of pain racing through my limbs and at least had the effect of diverting my attention from the distress of my stomach," Reston said. The needling was followed by moxibustion: two pieces of the herb wormwood were lit and held near the patient's abdomen. Reston immediately felt better.[4]

What unprecedented type of medicine is this? Acupuncture is "nothing marvelous,"[5] but it is pragmatic medicine based on thousands of years of application. It involves not only the use of needles inserted into special points on the body but also the use of massage (*an na*) and cauterization (moxibustion).[6] Acupuncture is the ancient Chinese art of healing, and like all Chinese arts and sciences, it has a philosophical basis. Only by understanding Taoist philosophy can one expect to understand acupuncture.

---

[4] "Yang, Yin and Needles," *Time*, XCVIII (August 9, 1971), 37.
[5] *Ibid.*, p. 38.
[6] Denis and Joyce Lawson-Wood, *The Five Elements of Acupuncture and Chinese Massage* (Russington, Sussex, England: Health Science Press, 1966), p. 23.

CHAPTER TWO

The Philosophy of Acupuncture

Yang and Yin

Five thousand to eight thousand years ago, the basic premise of Oriental philosophy was stated by the Chinese emperor Fu Hsi. This One Law declares: "The universe represents the interplay of the two activities, Yang and Yin, and their vicissitudes." Yang and Yin are opposites and thus attract each other. Their sum is Zero or Tao which produces and composes the world. All beings and phenomena in the universe are complex aggregates of Yang and Yin in varying proportions—nothing is entirely Yang nor entirely Yin. Hence all is in unceasing polarization and motion, and nothing in the universe is stable or finished. All beings and phenomena exist in a state of dynamic equilibrium. The harmonious existence of any individual being or circumstance depends on "the maintaining of the relative proportions of Yang and Yin appro-

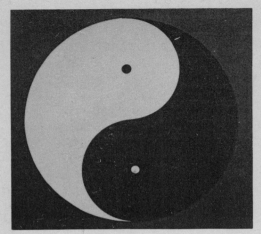

Figure 1. Yin-Yang, the two extremes.

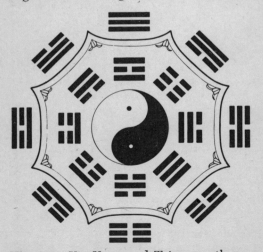

Figure 2. Yin-Yang and Trigrams, the symbols of the various combinations of Yang and Yin. Dashed lines represent Yin, and solid lines represent Yang. There are eight basic combinations or Trigrams.

Qualities

YANG FORCE	YIN FORCE
Plus	Minus
Light	Dark
Hot	Cold
Man	Woman
The urge to grow outward	The urge to shrink inward
Sol phase	Gel phase

Symptoms

YANG FORCE	YIN FORCE
Pain	Paralysis
Burning sensation	Cold
Spasms	Laxity
Overactivity	Underactivity
Excess	Deficiency

priate to the individual," the maintaining of dynamic balance.[1]

The essence of this philosophy lies in the nature of Yang and Yin. The urge *to grow outward* (Yang) and the urge *to shrink inward* (Yin) summarize the entire workings of the universe. Yang —the positive, the sunny side, the expanding or centrifugal force—complements Yin—the negative, the dark side, the diminishing or centripetal force. One force cannot exist without the other, and each implies its opposite. If Yang alone existed, there would be continuous, unimpeded expansion, gradually resulting in disappearance. Therefore this movement outward from the center must be balanced by a movement inward toward the center (Yin). On the other hand, if Yin alone existed, there would be a continuous diminishing to a point, or focusing to nothing. Hence Yang and Yin must coexist and balance each other for anything real to exist.

Ch'i and the Meridians

The human body, as well as the creation of the cosmos, is ordered by the interplay of Yang and Yin. The interaction of the two produces a vital energy. This bipolar energy is called *ch'i* and represents the life essence of the body. The English phrase *to be angry* is the equivalent of the Chinese phrase *to produce ch'i* to *die* equals *to stop ch'i* in Chinese. The breath of life or *ch'i* has three levels

[1] Lawson-Wood, *The Five Elements of Acupuncture and Chinese Massage, op. cit.*, pp. 15–16.

of manifestation in the body: deep, surface, and connecting. Anything affecting the *ch'i* on one level will affect every other level. One can cause a change in the body, for healing or for relieving pain, by skillfully influencing the *ch'i* surface level. The paths of energy on this level are called the meridians. Rebalancing of *ch'i* "as it circulates in the Inner Organs is effected by acupuncture treatment at certain surface points on the peripheral circuits known as the meridians."[2] There are twelve meridians related to specific internal organs, of which six are predominantly Yin and six predominantly Yang. The Yin meridians lie lower under the skin than the Yang. They are the meridians of the heart, the liver, the kidney, the spleen, the lung, and the pericardium (this last is actually the entire vascular system). The Yang meridians, running through the upper layers of the skin, control the stomach, the large intestine, the small intestine, the gallbladder, the bladder, and the triple heater (which regulates the body temperature and corresponds to the hypothalamus).[3] While the Yin meridians meet at the chest, the Yang meridians meet at the head. No single meridian maintains the same tissue depth throughout the entire body, but the distance between the meridian and the surface of the skin varies at each point.

In addition to the twelve organ meridians, there are the conceptional-vessel and the governor-vessel meridians. The conceptional-vessel meridian runs up the front center of the body, ending at a

[2] *Ibid.*, p. 53.
[3] *Ibid.*, p. 44.

ORGANS AND MERIDIANS

YANG FORCE

Stomach

Large intestine

Small intestine

Bladder

Gallbladder

Triple heater
(hypothalamus)

Meet at the head
running near surface of skin

ORGANS AND MERIDIANS

YIN FORCE

Heart

Liver

Kidneys

Spleen

Lungs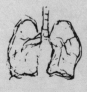

Pericardium
(vascular system)

Meet at the chest
running deeper under the skin

point between the two front teeth of the lower gum. This meridian can control all six of the Yin organ meridians. Points along its path have the power to influence the *ch'i* in the Yin organs. Since this meridian can engender change in other meridians, it is characterized as being conceptional. The governor-vessel meridian runs up the back center of the body and over the head, ending at a point between the two front teeth of the upper gum. Therefore, when the mouth is closed, the conceptional-vessel meridian and the governor-vessel meridian join in the mouth to bisect the entire body into left and right halves. The governor-vessel meridian governs the six Yang organ meridians. Together the two vessel meridians supplement and aid the other twelve meridians.

The flow of *ch'i* through the meridians is in a one-way direction only. There is never any flow in the opposite direction. It is the acupuncturist's task to restore the body's balance by reducing excess *ch'i* or by restoring deficient *ch'i*. However, the *ch'i* must be channeled in the one-way direction, and this involves the matter of five elements and cycles of flow.

The following illustrations, Figures 3 to 14, show the fourteen acupuncture meridians individually. Beside each acupuncture point is the Chinese character representing the point's name. Translation of the Chinese name into English does not reveal much about the uses of the point. Indeed, there is little direct relation between the name of the point and the efficacy of the point. For example, the second point of the lung meridian is named

雲 門 *or* Yun-men. *This is literally translated as Cloud Gate. Needling at* Yun-men *can relieve heart disease or chest pain; it does not have much to do with clouds or gates. The meaning of the name Cloud Gate is rooted in ancient Chinese history and philosophy. The Emperor of China who conferred the name Cloud Gate on this point had just won a great battle. In order to celebrate his glory, he led a victory march through the city gates. He commemorated his celestial triumph by naming the second point on the lung meridian Cloud Gate. Owing to the great antiquity of both Chinese acupuncture and Chinese history, the origins of most names have been lost. Only the names themselves remain, handed down from generations of acupuncturists.*

Figure 3.   The lung meridian,
         the large-intestine meridian

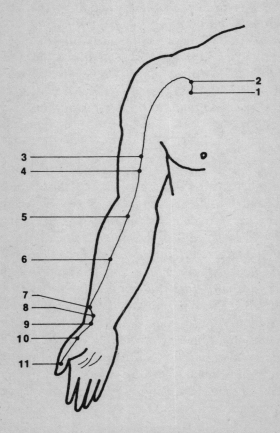

THE LUNG MERIDIAN

	CHINESE CHARACTERS	ROMANIZATION	LITERAL TRANSLATION
1.	中府	Chung fu	Center palace.
2.	雲門	Yün men	Cloud gate (flourishing).
3.	天府	T'ien fu	Celestial palace.
4.	俠白	Hsia pai	Pure white.
5.	尺澤	Ch'ih tse	One foot deep pool (small pool).
6.	孔最	K'ung tsui	Great extreme.
7.	列缺	Lieh ch'üeh	Lightening.
8.	經渠	Ching ch'ü	Past drain.
9.	太淵	T'ai yüan	Deep gulf.
10.	魚際	Yü chi	Fish border (meaty part of palm).
11.	少商	Shao shang	Less consult.

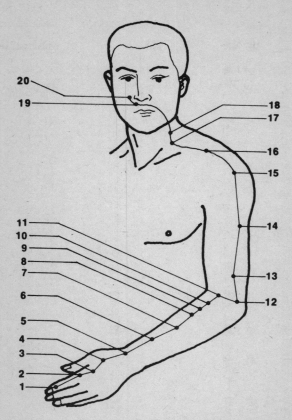

THE LARGE INTESTINE MERIDIAN

	CHINESE CHARACTERS	ROMANIZATION	LITERAL TRANSLATION
1.	商陽	Shang yang	Bright consult.
2.	二間	Erh chien	Second space.
3.	三間	San chien	Third space.

CHINESE CHARACTERS		ROMANIZATION	LITERAL TRANSLATION
4.	合谷	Ho ku	Joint valley.
5.	陽溪	Yang ch'i	Bright creek.
6.	偏歷	Pien li	Away from the point.
7.	溫溜	Wen liu	Warm to ramble.
8.	下廉	Hsia lien	Below space.
9.	上廉	Shang lien	Above space.
10.	三里	San li	Three miles.
11.	曲池	Ch'ü ch'ih	Crooked pool.
12.	肘髎	Chou chiao	Elbow bone.
13.	五里	Wu li	Five miles.
14.	臂臑	Pei nao	Forearm-ulna.
15.	肩髃	Chien yü	Shoulder bone.
16.	巨骨	Chü ku	Large bone.
17.	天鼎	T'ien ting	Heaven tripod.
18.	扶突	Fu t'u	Uphold suddenly.
19.	禾髎	Ho hsiao	Bone near nose.
20.	迎香	Ying hsiang	Welcome fragrance.

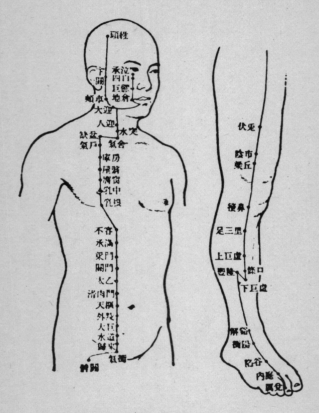

Figure 4. The stomach meridian.

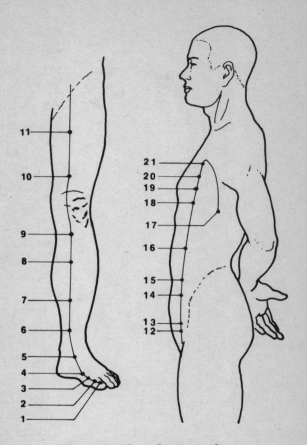

Figure 5. The spleen meridian.

	CHINESE CHARACTERS	ROMANIZATION	LITERAL TRANSLATION
1.	隱白	Yin pai	Hidden white.
2.	大都	Ta tou	Great capital.
3.	太白	T'ai pai	Whitest.

	CHINESE CHARACTERS	ROMANIZATION	LITERAL TRANSLATION
4.	公孫	Kung sun	Surname.
5.	商丘	Shang ch'iu	Small hill.
6.	三陰交	San yin chiao	Three "Yin" joint place.
7.	漏谷	Lou ku	Leaking valley.
8.	地機	Ti chi	Place of opportunity.
9.	陰陵泉	Yin ling ch'üan	Spring of "Yin" hill.
10.	血海	Hsüeh hai	Ocean of blood.
11.	箕門	Ch'i men	Wide door.
12.	衝門	Ch'ung men	Rush through.
13.	荷舍	Fu she	My home.
14.	腹結	Fu chieh	Knot in abdomen.
15.	大橫	Ta heng	Wide.
16.	腹哀	Fu ai	Abdomen grief.
17.	食竇	Shih tou	Concerning digestive organ.
18.	天溪	T'ien hsi	Mountain-stream.
19.	胸鄉	Hsiung hsiang	Chest area.
20.	周榮	Chou jung	Complete glory.
21.	大包	Ta pao	Big package.

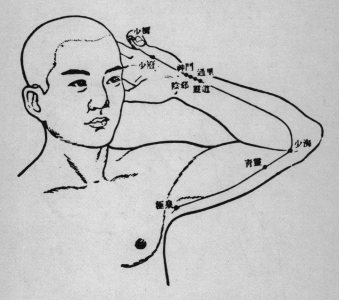

Figure 6. The heart meridian.

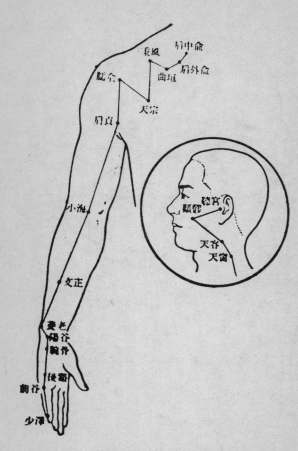

Figure 7. The small-intestine meridian.

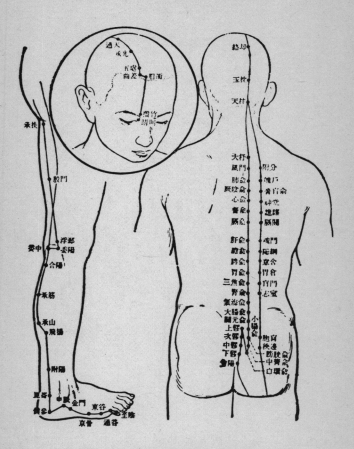

Figure 8. The bladder meridian.

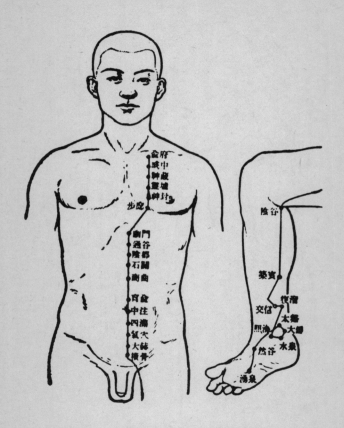

Figure 9. The kidney meridian.

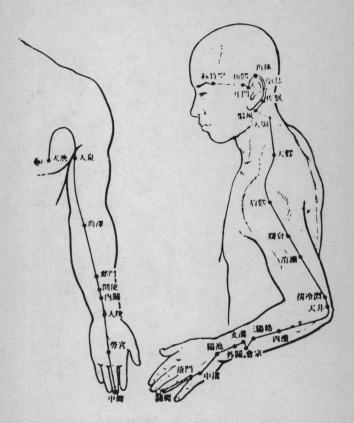

Figure 10. The pericardium (vascular system)
meridian (left).
The triple heater (hypothalamus)
meridian (right).

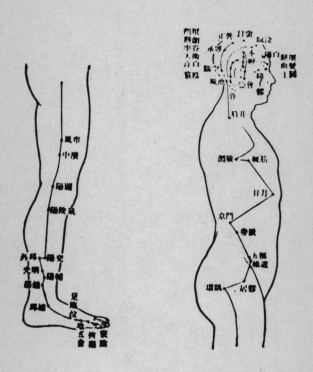

Figure 11. The gallbladder meridian.

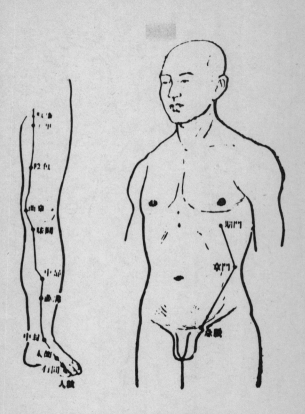

Figure 12. The liver meridian.

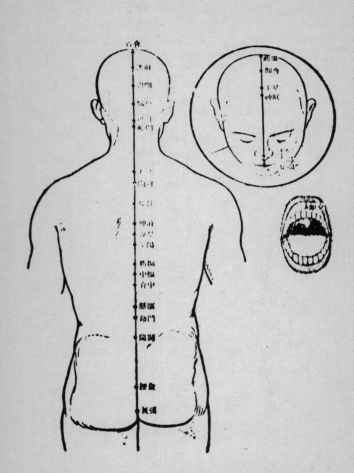

Figure 13. The governor-vessel meridian.

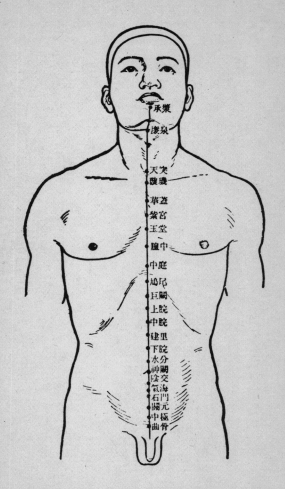

Figure 14. The conceptual-vessel meridian.

The following illustrations, Figures 15 to 21, show a combination of the acupuncture meridians on specific parts of the body. Instead of presenting each meridian individually as in the preceding group of figures, this group presents the meridians on an anatomical basis. All the meridians on the head are shown. All the meridians on the torso are shown. All the meridians on the arms and those on the legs are shown.

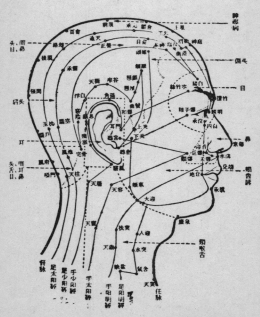

Figure 15. A view of the head with the meridians and acupuncture points.

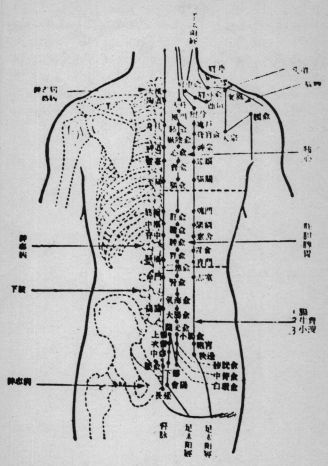

Figure 16. A back view of the torso with the
meridians and acupuncture points.

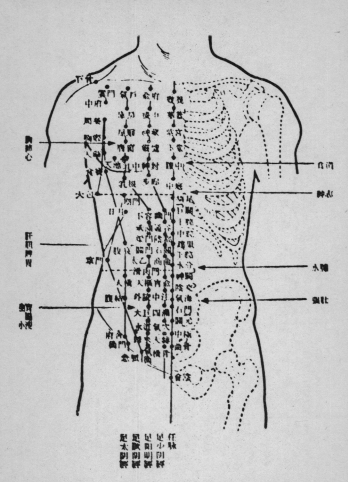

Figure 17. A front view of the torso with the meridians and acupuncture points.

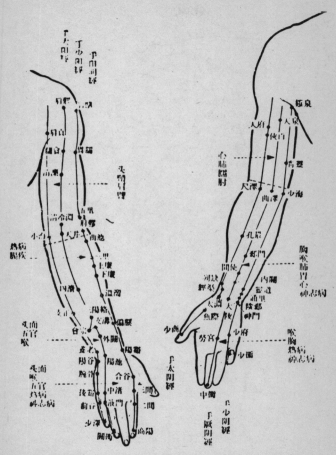

Figure 18. A view of the arms with the meridians and acupuncture points.

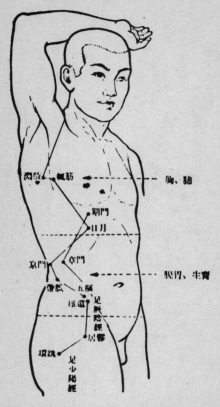

Figure 19. A side view of the torso with the meridians and acupuncture points.

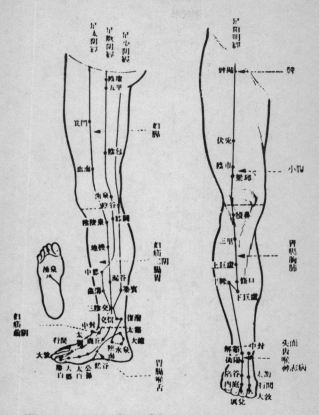

Figure 20. Inside and front views of the legs with the meridians and acupuncture points.

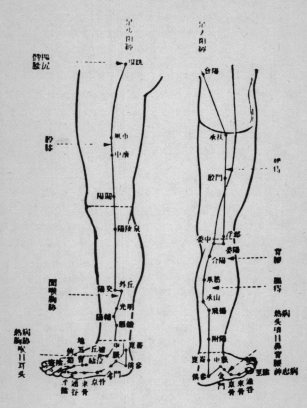

Figure 21. Outside and back views of the legs with the meridians and acupuncture points.

The Five Elements and Their Cycles

Briefly stated, the Taoist philosophers recognized the elements composing all creation to be wood, fire, earth, metal, water. Wood feeds fire. Fire begets earth in the form of ashes. Earth begets metal (ore). Metal is defined also as slime and air, slime being composed of earth and water. Hence metal begets water. Water, in turn, gives life to vegetation or wood. This is the *sheng* (generation) cycle, the cycle of a "mother-child relationship." Another cycle is the *k'o* (control) cycle of subjugation. Water extinguishes fire. Fire melts metal. Metal cuts wood. Wood subjugates earth (the wooden plow turns up the soil). Earth dams water. This cycle is star-shaped, and each element subdues the next but one.[4]

Each of the body's internal organs is associated with an element. Since the *sheng* and *k'o* cycles control the relation between elements, they also control the relations between internal organs. *Ch'i* flows only in the directions of these cycles—not in the opposite directions. For example, the heart is associated with the element of fire, the liver with wood, and the kidneys with water. If the heart is weak, it lacks *ch'i*. To supplement this lack, the acupuncturist can apply either of two methods. He can follow the *sheng* cycle and use a wood organ, like the liver, to "feed the fire" (stimulate the heart). Or he can directly needle the fire point along the heart meridian, achieving the same

[4] *Ibid.*, p. 45.

effect. (On each meridian there are acupuncture points corresponding to the five elements.) If the heart is overactive or has an excess of *ch'i*, the k'o cycle is used to correct this imbalance. A water organ (the kidneys) is manipulated by acupuncture to "put out the fire" and calm the heart. Or the water point along the heart meridian may be needled. Any imbalance of *ch'i*, causing spasms or laxity in any of the organs, can be corrected by the *sheng* or *k'o* cycles.

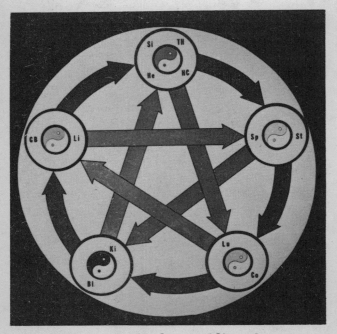

Figure 22. The *sheng* and *k'o* cycles.

CYCLES

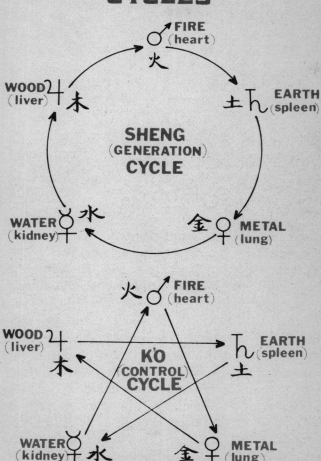

CHAPTER THREE

Acupuncture in Practice

The Point

The acupuncturist must decide into which of more than one thousand points he will insert the needle. Seven hundred thirty acupuncture points, with names like "Cloud Gate" and "Heavenly Palace," are familiar to all competent acupuncturists. These basic points lie on the meridians on opposite sides of the body, 365 on the left and the same number on the right. The extra points, which lie beyond the meridians, are known only to the masters of the art. The location of the acupuncture points does not generally correspond to the areas or organs of treatment. For example, the little toe is punctured to relieve a headache, the little finger for the heart troubles. The basic acupuncture points and the areas of treatment are, of course, joined by the meridians. In fact, Western doctors will concur that in the case of angina pectoris, commonly associated with heart diseases, the pain moves across the chest, down the arm, and terminates in the little finger. This is exactly the course of the heart meridian.[1]

There are many ways to locate the acupuncture points, although the ancients relied chiefly on the system of *ts'un* and *fen* measurements. One *ts'un* equals a "personal" inch. This is not the standardized inch equaling 2.54 centimeters. Rather, the *ts'un* is a personalized unit of measurement appropriate only to the patient himself. When the patient's middle finger is crooked, the distance from one joint wrinkle to the other is exactly one *ts'un*. The length across the four fingers of one hand (excluding the thumb) is three *ts'uns*, and from elbow to wrist it is twelve *ts'uns*. One *fen* equals one-tenth of a *ts'un* and often is used to indicate the depth to which a needle is inserted. Naturally, the *ts'un* varies minutely from individual to individual in the same proportion that the location of an acupuncture point varies. (The *ts'un-fen* system of measurement is far less arbitrary than the old British system, which decreed an inch to be three dried barleycorns laid end to end, and a rod to be the length of the left feet of the first sixteen men out of church.) By studying charts and by palpation, experienced practitioners can locate the points. In addition, there is a punctoscope, invented in 1963 by the French. This machine registers electrical microcurrents received through a searching pointer. When the pointer is led over the hand, at a certain point a red light

[1] Eileen Simpson, "Acupuncture (à la française)," *Saturday Review*, LV (February 19, 1972), 48.

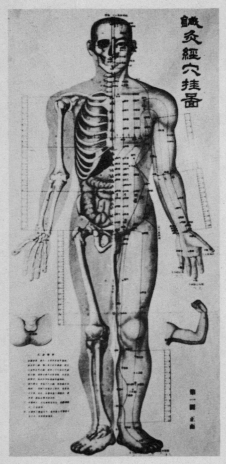

Figure 23. The *ts'un-fen* measurements and the meridians on the front of the body.

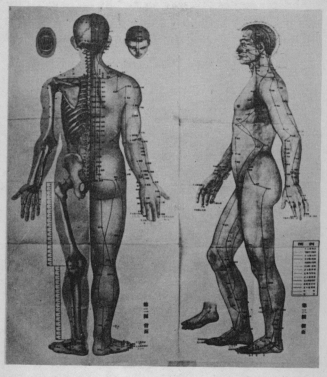

Figure 24. The *ts'un-fen* measurements and the meridians on the back and side of the body.

indicating electrical current will glow. This point on the hand is an acupuncture point.[2] The punctoscope can locate a point to within one-tenth of a millimeter, unless there is a cut or an insect bite on the skin, for these openings let out the *ch'i*. Therefore no traditional acupuncturist would allow himself to use this machine.

Needling

By far the most conspicuous (and, to some, the most frightening) aspect of acupuncture is the needle. Needles vary in length from half an inch to ten inches[3] or more. They range in diameter from hair-fine to very thick. They have been composed of many materials—stone, wood, bone—but mostly metal. The gold and platinum needles have a Yang force and are used to stimulate and strengthen. Silver needles have a Yin force and are used for relaxing and soothing. There is the five- (or seven-) star needle, a hammer-like instrument with many short needles affixed to its head. This is often tapped on children or weak adults. Most modern acupuncturists employ the efficient stainless steel needle for a majority of treatments. Unlike the gold, platinum, and silver needles, the stainless steel needle does not have a predetermined Yang or Yin force. Its force and the effect it will have depend on how it is manipulated. This may

[2] Henriette Chandet, "Les Aiguilles Mystérieuses," *Paris Match*, No. 1190 (February 26, 1972), 60.
[3] "A Prickly Panacea Called Acupuncture," *Life*, LXXI (August 13, 1972), 33.

be explained by the fact that stainless steel is an alloy, whereas the other metals are pure.

Inserting the needle is rather involved, for there are many steps. The acupuncturist must first locate the most effective acupuncture point. He must then determine the angle of insertion. After piercing the skin with the needle, the acupuncturist must insert the needle to the proper depth. The needle must be left in place for the proper length of time. The insertion may be a simple in-and-out motion, or it may involve rotation. While the other fingers control the angle and force of the needle, the forefinger and thumb rotate it clockwise or counterclockwise. In a man (considered mostly a Yang being) clockwise rotation stimulates while counterclockwise rotation calms. In a woman (considered mostly a Yin being) the reverse is true. The Sparrow-peck method is a rapid in-and-out motion of the needle while the needle's point remains below the surface of the skin. The needle may be inserted and left in the body for several minutes, sometimes for days. While left in the body, it may be tapped or vibrated in order to stimulate the organs.

The most common angle of insertion is ninety degrees. In acupuncture it is important that the needle go deep enough into the skin. Where the skin is thick, this is best accomplished at an angle of ninety degrees. Around the face and head, the angle of insertion is usually forty-five degrees. Thirty- and fifteen-degree insertions are also used. In most cases the puncture is bloodless, although for stroke or swollen arthritis cases, blood is inten-

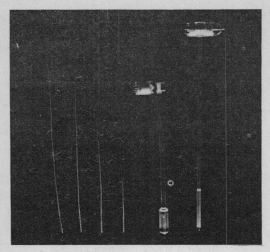

Figure 25. Gold needles and five- and seven-star needles.

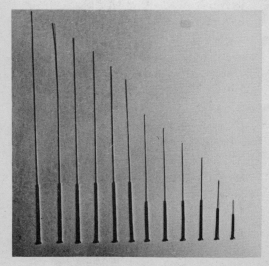

Figure 26. Silver needles.

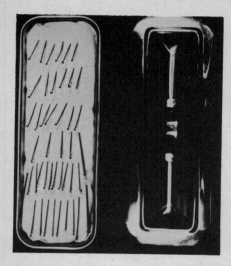

Figure 27.
Stainless
steel needles.

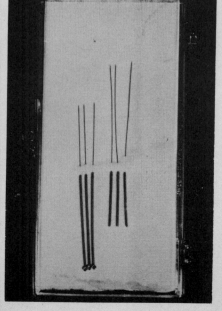

Figure 28.
Very fine
stainless
steel needles.

tionally let out. There is no opening in acupuncture needles to trap blood and to pass it on to other patients. Indeed, infection is very rare. Sterilization is usually performed in alcohol, sometimes in steam or in autoclaves or gas sterilizers.

The needle has no therapeutic value in itself, but serves merely as a conductor. It transmits the

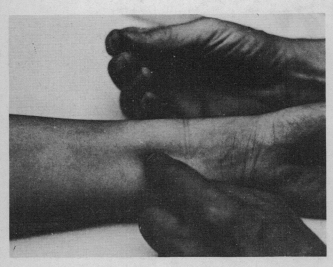

Figure 29. Locating the point.

energy (*ch'i*) from the doctor's body into the patient at the acupuncture point. This action re-opens the blocked passage of *ch'i* and allows a re-balancing of vital energy. However, this can also be accomplished by the other methods of acupuncture: *an na* (loosely called massage) and moxibustion.

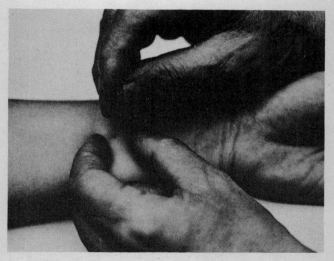

Figure 30. Inserting the needle.

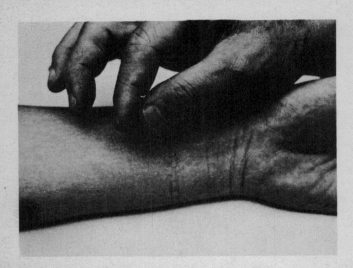

Figure 31. Rotating the needle.

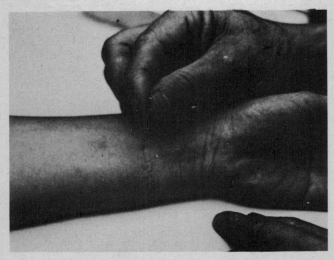

Figure 32. Rotating the needle.

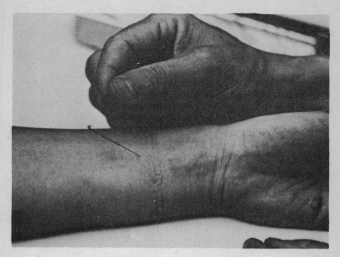

Figure 33. Forty-five-degree angle of insertion.

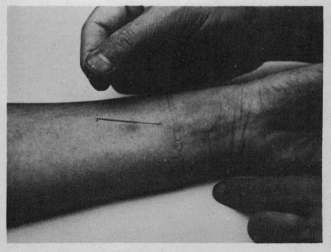

Figure 34. Fifteen-degree angle of insertion.

An Na and Ai

"Massage" or *an na* consists of a prolonged concentration of pressure at an acupuncture point. This focusing of force has the same result as needling but without the needle. In ancient times *an na* was practiced with the hands, long before needles. *An na* techniques now include the use of a special instrument (an ivory or bone needle ending in a ball), the use of the fingers, fingernail, knuckles, and elbows. Pressure, friction, movement, and percussion are achieved by these various techniques. The traditional massage instrument, which must be a nonconductor, is rubbed with light, rapid, unidirectional force on the skin. This causes a small electrical charge to build up, which will eventually discharge itself at a point of low resistance. It has been demonstrated that the acupuncture points coincide with small areas of high conductivity or low electrical resistance. Any static charge will therefore have an effect on the body by penetrating through the acupuncture points to the internal organs.[4]

In addition to needles and *an na*, acupuncturists employ moxibustion. The herb involved in this treatment is dried wormwood (*Artemesia*) called *ai*. After the leaves have been ground and aged for several years, the herb looks like gray-brown wool. A small conical clump of *ai* is held near the acupuncture point or molded onto the

[4] Denis and Joyce Lawson-Wood, *The Five Elements of Acupuncture and Chinese Massage* (Russington, Sussex, England: Health Science Press, 1966), p. 74.

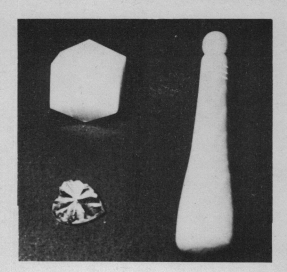

Figure 35. *An na* instruments.

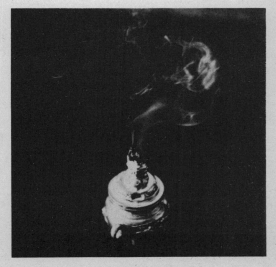

Figure 36. Burning *ai*.

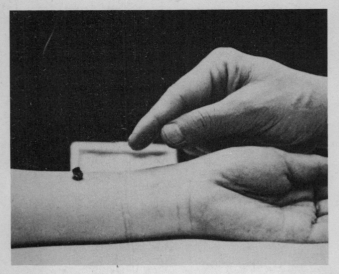

Figure 37. Moxibustion.

handle of an inserted needle or placed beside an inserted needle. The herb is then lit, giving off a pungent odor, and its great heat stimulates the body and increases the Yang. Since *moxa* adds energy, it is usually practiced on paralytics and stroke patients, or used during the winter.

These then are the techniques of acupuncture, performed only after a thorough diagnosis.

Diagnosis—the True Art

Before the acupuncturist can take a single therapeutic action, he must have a thorough understanding of the illness. Diagnosis is perhaps the great art of acupuncture, and it is diagnosis that one must master if one wishes to be more than a mere technician. Although a four-step formula exists, these steps are far from foolproof and depend on personal judgment. The initial step is (1) to *look*—look at the patient's color, bearing, eyes, and tongue. Then (2) *listen*, to his heart, voice, and breathing. The next step places the patient-doctor relationship on a very personal level: the doctor must (3) *ask* the patient everything that could possibly affect his mind, spirit and, hence, body. From what the patient eats to what he feels about the cosmos, the doctor should cover a range of questions. Finally, the fourth and hardest step is (4) to *take the pulse*. This is indeed a matter of skill, patience, and talent. The acupuncturist who is in ill health may just as well heal himself first, for he cannot correctly take a pulse. Absolute silence, a relaxed patient, and a calmly receptive doctor are essential since the pulses are so complex. There are six pulses on each wrist, and each pulse may have as many as twenty-seven characteristics.[5] Three fingers (index, middle, and fourth) are placed on the wrist, with the middle finger resting on the prominence of the wrist bone and the index finger nearest the hand. The practitioner always uses his left fingers on the patient's right wrist and vice versa. On the right wrist there are six pulses, three of which (large intestine, stomach, and triple heater) are detected with light pressure of the

[5] "A Prickly Panacea Called Acupuncture," p. 34.

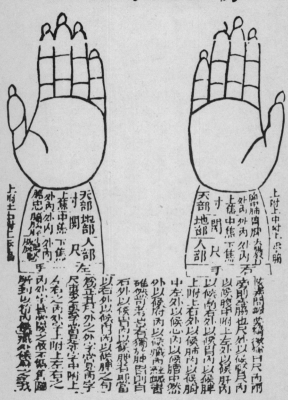

Figure 38. A diagram of the pulses. Reproduced from the *Golden Mirror*, an encyclopedia, containing the early medical writings of the Han dynasty (206 B.C.–220 A.D.), compiled under the edict of the emperor K'ang Hsi (1661–1722 A.D.).

PULSES

YANG FORCE	YIN FORCE
Small intestine	Heart
Gallbladder	Liver
Bladder	Kidneys
Large intestine	Lungs
Stomach	Spleen
Triple heater (hypothalamus)	Circulation (pericardium)

fingers and three (lungs, spleen, and circulation organ) with heavy pressure. Light pressure on the left hand gives the pulses of small intestine, gallbladder, and bladder; heavy pressure gives the pulses of heart, liver, and kidneys. The light or superficial pulses on both hands are all Yang organ pulses. The heavy-pressure pulses correspond to pulses of Yin organs. Pulse taking can last for fifteen to twenty minutes, which is still a short time when one remembers that the ancient Chinese often listened for hours. The Chinese preferred one hour of diagnosis and thirty seconds of treatment to thirty seconds of diagnosis followed by an hour of treatment.[6] Not only can the practitioner discover the individual health of each organ and their combined functioning, but he can also detect, to a

[6] Lawson-Wood, *op. cit.*, p. 65.

certain quantitative degree, the high or low blood pressure of the entire organism. A harmonious rhythm of the pulses indicates the body's well-being.

The Practitioner Himself

The doctor's individuality and judgment are more important in Oriental than in Western medicine. In most cases, professional discretion causes the acupuncturist to experiment with any methods of needling first on himself, before he dares to practice on his patient. He will always explain his actions and their possible effects beforehand, warning the patient of any sensations he might feel. Acupuncture treatment is very personalized, and the diagnostic "talking it out" helps the patient as well as the doctor. All treatments, like all patients, are unique; for the same illness there are varying cures. The main acupuncture points and combinations are flexible—for each according to his need. Because the Orientals believe that the spirit and the body are inseparable, the treatment to cure the body must take into account the individual spirit.

Such philosophical beliefs guarantee that most acupuncturists are men of high ideals and dedication. A diligent acupuncturist will think nothing of long· hours and hard work. Such a practitioner solicits no business, nor will he accept a patient without the recommendation of a former patient. It is the humanitarian spirit which characterizes his practice, and he considers his calling to be unlike any other business—something different, special—for human life is involved.

A certain Los Angeles acupuncturist has helped persons ranging in age from five months to ninety-eight years. It is interesting to note that the female patient is markedly less afraid of the needle than the male. Not only are the women patients braver, but they also stand pain better. The pain that spreads through the body from the acupuncture back point is like an "electric shock." Most of those ailing suffer from bursitis or backaches; 80 percent of these do not require a third treatment for recovery, and 50 percent need only one treatment.

However, it is important to note that recovery times are individualized. With one person a disease is healed at once; with another the same disease is healed only after several treatments. Acupuncture is more than self-hypnosis and cannot be explained on a merely psychosomatic basis. Therefore it is not surprising to learn that the patient's mental attitude (enthusiastic or suspicious) does not determine the recovery period. However, race, personal habits, and food do make a difference in reaction to acupuncture—all of which stresses acupuncture's physiological aspects.

CHAPTER FOUR

From the Stone Age Onward

Acupuncture has come down through many millennia of Chinese folk medicine. Allegedly discovered when soldiers wounded by arrows found their other ailments improving,[1] acupuncture was popular as early as the Stone Age. In the primitive pre-metal society the *pien* ("sharp stone") was used to cure diseases by pricking or pressing. This was later replaced by needles of stone, bone, bamboo and, eventually, of copper, iron, silver, and gold. About five thousand years ago the *Nei Ching* (*Book of Internal Medicine*) was written. This is the earliest extant medical classic in China, summing up all of Chinese medicine from the beginning of Chinese history. This classic must have been the textbook which enabled Pien Ch'üeh

[1] "A Prickly Panacea Called Acupuncture," *Life*, LXXI (August 13, 1972), 32.

to accomplish the first recorded acupuncture cure two thousand five hundred years ago; acupuncture was used to revive a dying man already in a coma.[2]

The *Nei Ching* contains sections dealing with "channels" and "points" on the body, needles and applications, diseases and ailments curable by acupuncture, and prohibitions (certain points forbidden to moxibustion or acupuncture, and the maximum depths of needle insertion). A later work (*Chen Chiu Chia I Ching—An Introduction to Acupuncture and Moxibustion*) listed 649 points on the human body. Since its compilation around 250 A.D. this book has had great influence in China and abroad. Progress in acupuncture increased in China until the mid-seventeenth century; a special acupuncture department was established in the Imperial Medical School in Peking (ca. 800 A.D.), the functions of points were clarified, and effective methods were discovered and taught. However, development was stifled in the Ch'ing or Manchurian Dynasty (1644–1911) by a ban on acupuncture practice. In an attempt to Westernize China, certain chief medical officials extended this ban to include all of Chinese medicine. This decree was largely ignored by the rural people in remote areas.[3]

With the Civil War and Communist supremacy, acupuncture entered an entirely new stage. Mao Tse-tung realized the enormity of any effort to retrain China's 500,000 traditional practitioners

---

[2] *Acupuncture Anaesthesia* (Peking: Foreign Languages Press, 1972), pp. 20–21.

[3] *Ibid.*, pp. 21–23.

into Western doctors.[4] At the same time he recognized that "Chinese medicine and pharmacology are a great treasure-house; efforts should be made to explore them and raise them to a higher level." Chinese medicine took a new and fortunate direction, and doctors were exhorted to "give both Chinese and Western treatment." Since 1949 there have been tremendous advances in acupuncture owing to the research in Peking hospitals and in other cities and provinces. The improvements in needles (longer, hot or warm, extra-fine, electrically activated) and the new methods of instruction and practice (instruments for locating meridians, porcelain figures marked with points) have been notable, but these take only second place in the advance of acupuncture. For what has first startled the Western world is acupuncture anesthesia. The anesthetic aspect of acupuncture was originally noticed when medical workers sought to relieve postoperative pain, especially in tonsillectomies. The good results led to the question, "Why can't acupuncture needling stop pain during operations as well as afterward?" Acupuncture was first used as a method of anesthesia in dentistry. Later its use was broadened to include all surgical procedures. From 1968 to 1971, acupuncture was used as the method of anesthesia in over 400,000 operations in China.[5]

[4] "Yang, Yin and Needles," *Time*, XCVIII (August 9, 1971), 38.
[5] *Acupuncture Anaesthesia*, pp. 24–25.

CHAPTER FIVE

Safe,
Simple,
Economical—
Acupuncture
Anesthesia

Such a development as acupuncture anesthesia is unprecedented in medical history. Those who have developed it say that it has been achieved by "combining new zeal with scientific approach, applying modern scientific knowledge and methods, and summing up and improving on the experience of traditional Chinese medicine." [1] Acupuncture anesthesia does not require complicated apparatus and is applicable in any climate, regardless of equipment and geographical conditions. Hence it is perfectly suitable for remote areas or war conditions. More importantly, the patient is fully conscious during the operation and can give play to his subjective healing role, responding to the surgeon's questions and taking a part in his own cure. In Western operations to correct squint-

[1] *Acupuncture Anaesthesia*, p. 1.

ing, the outcome is learned only after the anesthetic drug wears off. With acupuncture the patient can voluntarily move his eyes, and the surgeon can ascertain the results before the operation ends. During a thyroidectomy, the patient may respond to the surgeon's questions. This helps the surgeon to prevent damage to the nerves controlling the vocal chords. A patient undergoing orthopedic surgery retains the movement of his limbs. His active cooperation helps the doctor find the injured muscles and tendons easily. Furthermore, in plastic surgery, the patient can immediately test his new prosthesis before leaving the operating room.[2]

Acupuncture is a preferable form of anesthesia since it is free of toxic side effects. All conventional anesthetic drugs are "toxic to a point" and therefore pose potential hazards to the system.[3] In terms of the Western drugs, general anesthetic agents render the patient unconscious to pain—until he wakes up. Then the toxic side effects take their toll. The possible "hangover" of nausea, vomiting, weakness, and dizziness may last for several hours. Acupuncture prevents all this. In fact, it sets in motion and strengthens the body's functions since it plays the dual role of anesthetic and healing. Infections of the respiratory tract, pneumonia, and other complications which may follow inhalation anesthesia are also eliminated by acupuncture. Blood pressure, pulse, and breathing are normal during the operation. However, what most amazes West-

[2] *Ibid.*, pp. 2–3.
[3] "Nixon M.D. Acclaims Acupuncture," *Star-News*, April 12, 1972, p. 5.

ern physicians is the patient's mobility and normal activity. The patient can move about, eat food easily during the operation, and take tea with the doctors after the operation. For patients with poorly functioning livers, kidneys, or lungs, those with high blood pressure, or those suffering from shock or oversensitivity to drugs, acupuncture is often the safest anesthetic. In fact, acupuncture reduces the danger of shock, which is often deadlier than any fracture or wound. Effective, safe, simple, and economical—acupuncture anesthesia is claimed to be 90 percent successful.[4]

Under the Communist regime, acupuncture anesthesiologists have made great advances. The mortality rate after brain surgery has markedly decreased now that 90 percent of such surgery is done with acupuncture. A few years ago, only the body and ears were needled. Now the face and nose are also areas of needling. Instead of hand-rotated needles, the anesthesiologists have developed electrically vibrated needles. The needle shaft is connected by fine wires to a transistor which vibrates the needle rhythmically several hundred times per minute. In addition, streams of distilled water directed at the points of insertion have eliminated any unevenness that resulted from hand manipulation.[5] Prior to recent advances a pneumonectomy patient was needled at several dozen points—often more than a hundred—and four acupuncturists were needed to manipulate the needles continuously. Research has reduced the number of

[4] *Acupuncture Anaesthesia*, p. 3.
[5] *Ibid.*, pp. 25–26.

points to three, and in more than ninety thoracic operations only one needle is necessary.[6]

Before the patient even prepares for the operation, he is informed of the entire proces and advised of problems that might arise so that he can consciously help the surgeons.[7] There is no attempt to "push" acupuncture, however. The decision to use it as an anesthetic rests entirely with the patient. It would not be fair to subject a tense, frightened patient to consciousness during surgery. In such a case, general anesthesia is used.[8] The night before the operation, a sedative (such as four hundred milligrams of meprobamate) is given. During the operation, meperidine hydrochloride in fifty- to sixty-milligram doses may be given. In most instances acupuncture alone is sufficient. The needles are first inserted into the appropriate points, after which a small clip is attached to the needle shaft and a connection is made to a battery-powered unit. The patient, conscious and alert, begins to feel a combined swelling, soreness, heaviness, and numbness—the anesthesia has taken effect. Usually it takes twenty minutes for acupuncture to produce anesthesia. Throughout the operation the anesthetist carefully observes all the usual measurements and converses with the patient, who gives guidance as to the need for additional anesthetics. The intensity of anesthesia is greatest at the specific surgical site selected; however, there

[6] *Ibid.*, p. 6.
[7] *Ibid.*, p. 2.
[8] E. Gray Dimond, M.D., "Acupuncture Anesthesia," *The Journal of the American Medical Association*, CCXVIII (December 6, 1971), 1561.

is a generalized increase in pain tolerance throughout the entire body. This is useful if the surgeon must suddenly attend to another area of the body, since he can proceed without administering further anesthesia. At the commencement of surgery there is an initial "level" of pain. Once anesthesia for this "level" has been achieved, the anesthetic agent may be lessened. At certain less painful points during the operation the electrical stimulation of the needle is reduced to the minimum. Later the stimulation is increased as it is needed.[9] In this way, adequate anesthesia can be maintained indefinitely. After one brain tumor operation lasting for six hours, anesthesia persisted for several hours after withdrawal of the needles.[10]

The patients under acupuncture anesthesia are free to sip tea, as in the case of one undergoing brain surgery, or eat fruit, as in the case of a lobectomy patient. The surgical staff can rest and discuss the patient's progress in mid-operation. After the operation, many patients can sit up, step to the floor, and walk out.

[9] *Ibid.*, p. 1562.
[10] *Acupuncture Anaesthesia*, p. 17.

CHAPTER SIX

The Oriental Science in the Occident

An awareness of acupuncture has only very recently reached the West—or so it seems. For indeed the Jesuits of France, as early as the seventeenth century, brought back reports of acupuncture healing. In fact, Englebert Kaempfer, in a doctoral thesis in 1694, described the Japanese use of acupuncture and *moxa*.[1] Yet acupuncture remained a mystery to Western medicine until 1927, when Soulié de Morant, a French diplomat to Peking, demonstrated techniques to a French medical group and wrote a book, *Précis de la Vraie Acuponcture*. Today Paris is the Occidental center of this Oriental art. There are seven hundred physicians practicing acupuncture in France. The

[1] See John S. Bowers, and Robert W. Carubba, "The Doctoral Thesis of Engelbert Kaempfer: on Tropical Diseases, Oriental Medicine, and Exotic Natural Phenomenon," unpublished monograph, Pennsylvania State University.

Institut du Centre d'Acuponcture de France conducts a three-year acupuncture course. Naturally the European philosophy of healing lies within the scientific framework, necessitating medical-school training. Pulse readings are regarded as insufficient for diagnosis and are supplemented by x-ray and laboratory studies.[2]

In surveying the periodical references on acupuncture in a medical bibliography, one is impressed by the status of acupuncture in the modern medical world (notably outside of the United States). Both the Russians and the Czechoslovakians have done extensive research on acupuncture—from "The Efficacy of Acupuncture of the Shoulder Girdle Zone in the Treatment of Insomnia" to "Vasomotor Reactions Following Acupuncture in Lumbro-Sacral Syndromes." The French, Germans, Italians, Portuguese, and Rumanians have also observed and practiced. The Indonesians and Malaysians, as well as the Chinese, have published their findings and impressions in medical journals. Yet the majority of such medical reports do not deal with the reasons for acupuncture's efficacy. Why does it work?

[2] Eileen Simpson, "Acupuncture (à la française)," *Saturday Review,* LV (February 19, 1972), 48.

CHAPTER SEVEN

Why
Does
It
Work?

The imbalance of vital energy, the concept of Yang and Yin, and the Taoist philosophical reasons do not satisfy Western scientific minds. Perhaps acupuncture affects the nerve impulses or stimulates the supply of blood to the nerves.[1] There was evidence of a neural pathway when a procaine injection at an acupuncture point did not produce anesthesia at the distant site but did infiltrate around the acupuncture point and blocked the anesthetizing effect.[2] Furthermore, two scientists, Dr. Ronald Melzack of Canada and Dr. Patrick Wall of London, maintain that acupuncture needles "switch off certain pathways of pain" in the human body. The sensation of touch is conveyed to the brain by way of the large-nerve-fiber system, while the sensation of pain is conveyed by the way of the small-nerve-fiber system. A gate control cell in the

[1] Simpson, "Acupuncture (à la française)," p. 49.
[2] Dimond, "Acupuncture Anesthesia," p. 1563.

nerve system "switches" sensations from one fiber to another. When an acupuncture needle is inserted in a certain part of the body, it can "close the gate" and "switch off" the pain.[3] Further reports from the Russian Laboratory of Reflex Therapy are as yet inconclusive. Yet they show that acupuncture affects parasympathetic areas of the autonomic nervous system [4]—that part of the nervous system which stimulates secretions, slows heart movement, and dilates blood vessels. In attempting to explain the power of healing, some persons will consider only the emotional factors. They label acupuncture "psychosomatic medicine" and "self-hypnosis." [5] However, French experiments on laboratory animals have shown (though again the evidence is inconclusive) that acupuncture cannot be attributed to mere suggestion or a placebo effect. When a physician asked the head of the French Institut du Centre d'Acuponcture, "How many of your cures are attributable to suggestion?" the reply was, "About the same percentage as you have in your practice." [6]

In 1963 an article by a North Korean biologist appeared to be the first major breakthrough in the explanation of acupuncture. Kim Bong-han claimed that he had isolated the vital energy (ch'i) system by the classical methods of tissue staining and microscopy and by the use of radioactive tracers. The ch'i system was said to be composed of cor-

---

[3] Michael Cusack, "Acupuncture—Is Getting the Needle Good for You?", Science World, XXIV (May 15, 1972), 9.
[4] Simpson, op. cit., p. 49.
[5] "Yang, Yin and Needles," Time, XCVIII (August 9, 1971), 38.
[6] Simpson, loc. cit.

puscles grouped around acupuncture sites and ducts through which an acellular, but microscopically observable, fluid circulates. This discovery, although lauded by the North Koreans, is not acceptable to Western scientists.[7] A team of scientists and medical workers sent by the Communist Chinese to North Korea in order to check the report were unable to confirm the findings.[8]

Certainly the most promising explanation of acupuncture is one related to electrical charges in the body. Recently at the University of Syracuse, a specialist in skin grafting, Professor Robert Becker, M.D., was attempting to measure the electrical currents running through the human skin. He could not have been less interested in acupuncture. However, he discovered electrical circuits on the skin corresponding to the Chinese meridians. The French microvoltmeter (cantoni) shows that acupuncture points have greater electrical conductivity than the skin areas surrounding them. The Japanese have shown the same result along the meridians.[9] The Chinese researchers have used electrophysiological techniques on rabbits and by pain stimulation have produced a standard "induction voltage" in the cerebral cortex. Acupuncture lowered the cerebral induction voltage markedly even though the pain stimulation remained unchanged. Needling done on the ear produces anesthesia in the abdominal region. One study now in progress seems to identify nerve endings in the ear which,

---

[7] Dimond, *loc. cit.*
[8] *Ibid.*
[9] Simpson, *loc. cit.*

when stimulated, change the electrical resistance over the abdomen.[10]

A consideration of the colloidal-electrical theory may throw some light on the matter. Vital energy (*ch'i*) may be thought of as representing some form of electricity. It is not equivalent, but many of the laws applicable to one may be applicable to the other. A colloid is a suspension of very fine particles of one material in another medium. Mists, smokes, and emulsions are good examples of colloidal behavior. There are two phases in every colloid—the tendency of the particles to repel each other and spread (*sol* phase) and the tendency to coalesce and join together (*gel* phase). Without much imagination, one can easily equate the *sol* phase with Yang and the *gel* phase with Yin. It is scientifically accepted that life exists only where there is "protoplasm behaving colloidally"—or life represents the interplay of the two phases *gel* and *sol*. All colloids, especially living colloids, are electrically sensitive. An organism is composed of a complexity of colloidal structures, and any factor capable of changing colloidal behavior will have a significant effect on the entire organism.[11]

The Russian scientist Alfred Korzybski first formulated (ca. 1921) the importance of colloidal behavior. All drugs base their effect on colloidal equilibrium, for it is a fact that various acids or

[10] Dimond, *loc. cit.*
[11] Denis and Joyce Lawson-Wood, *The Five Elements of Acupuncture and Chinese Massage* (Russington, Sussex, England: Health Science Press, 1966), pp. 68–70.

alkalis change the electrical conductivity of proto-plasm. All illnesses are somehow related to col-loidal disturbances, and physical colloidal states are closely related to nervous and mental states. The factors which affect colloidal behavior, hence the entire well-being of an organism, are physical factors (light, heat, electricity, all radiant energy), biological factors (microbes, parasites), chemical factors (drugs, poisons), and mechanical factors (friction, puncture, pressure, sonic waves). There-fore, it is clear that needling and *an na* (both mechanical factors) and moxibustion (a physical factor) are of healing value because of their ability to alter colloidal behavior.[12]

[12] *Ibid.*, pp. 70–72.

CHAPTER EIGHT

What Acupuncture Can Cure: The Physiological Illness

If one accepts the validity of the collodial theory, one can conclude that acupuncture is capable of curing or alleviating most diseases arising from physiological abnormalities, in which colloidal equilibrium is upset. This seems to be true. Acupuncture cannot heal permanent scars or lesions. It cannot rejuvenate worn-out organs, but it can regulate them for better efficiency and functioning. It is no longer used for treatment of infectious diseases like cholera, for antibiotics have replaced it; but it dissipates the disagreeable effects of such diseases.[1] The effect of acupuncture is most evident on various types of paralysis and neuralgia: on epilepsy, migraine, toothache, tonsillitis, hyper-acidity of the stomach, gastralgia, intestinal ca-

[1] Eileen Simpson, "Acupuncture (à la française)," *Saturday Review*, LV (February 19, 1972), 48.

tarrh, intestinal cramps, indigestion, inflammation
of the bladder and urinary tract, gonorrhea, bron-
chitis, rheumatic inflammation of the joints, men-
strual difficulties, complications in childbirth, eye
inflammation, allergy, irritation, glaucoma, cata-
ract, ringing in the ears, rashes, excessive perspira-
tion,[2] diarrhea, worms and parasites, constipation,
emphysema, frigidity, impotence, and nervous de-
pression.[3] Acupuncture treatments have had effects
on multiple sclerosis, frostbite,[4] appendicitis,[5] peritonitis,[6] insomnia,[7] asthma,[8] poliomyelitis,[9] and
massive hemorrhaging.[10] Furthermore, acupuncture
is claimed to have healing power over deafness. A
lay medical practitioner in the Kirin province of
China, Chao Pu-yu, experimented by inserting the

[2] Dana Heroldová. *Acupuncture and Moxibustion* (New York:
Altai Press, 1968), p. 80.
[3] Henriette Chandet, "Les Aiguilles Mystérieuses," *Paris Match*,
No. 1190 (February 26, 1972), p. 60.
[4] See C. Ch'en, "Acupuncture in the Treatment of Frostbite,"
Zhong hua Waike Zazhi, VII (October, 1959), 1031.
[5] See "Acupuncture and Traditional Drugs in the Treatment of
Appendicitis: Analysis of 49 cases," *Chinese Medical Journal*,
LXIX (July, 1959), 62–66.
[6] See T. H. Wu, "Acupuncture in the Treatment of Generalized
Peritonitis," *Zhong hua Waike Zazhi*, VII (December, 1959),
1193–1195.
[7] See L. M. Klimenko, "The Efficacy of Acupuncture of the
Shoulder Girdle Zone in the Treatment of Insomnia," *Vracheb-
noe Delo*, X (October, 1969), 126–127.
[8] See E. A. Udovitskaia, "Treatment of Bronchial Asthma
Patients by the Acureflexotherapy Method," *Vrachebnoe Delo*,
XI (November, 1969), 128–130.
[9] See S. C. Jen, "Acupuncture in the Treatment of Paralytic
Poliomyelitis," *Paediatrica Indoneseiana*, V Supplement (July–
December, 1965), 699–702.
[10] See Y. K. Ch'ien *et al.*, "Experimental Studies on Acu-
puncture in the Therapy of Massive Hemorrhage," *Zhong hua
Waike Zazhi*, XI (1963), 377–378.

needle at a prohibitive depth in the base of his own skull. The resulting sensation was so powerful that his numbed hand could hardly twist the needle. The sensation combined a feeling of congestion in the neck, a burning throat, and limbs numbed as though by an electric shock. These effects had been proved successful in earlier treatments and proved successful in the healing of persons deaf and mute from childhood illnesses. Of the 168 deaf-mute children in the school at Liaoyuan, Kirin, 157 regained their hearing and 149 could begin to speak. This "miracle" occurred three years ago, and the treatment is now widespread throughout China.[11] A certain acupuncturist in the United States has given a young boy twelve treatments for deafness. During this time the child's hearing has increased by 25 percent.

[11] "The Mutes Regain Their Speech," *China Reconstructs*, XXI (February, 1972), 8–9.

CHAPTER NINE

Not
Magic

Acupuncture is definitely not a medical marvel with unlimited curative powers. For some illnesses it heals, for others it does not help at all, and in other cases it just lessens some of the symptoms.[1] Like any therapy, it also has its weaknesses. The use of acupuncture anesthesia is still to be perfected. At certain stages during an operation, patients may feel discomfort when internal organs are pulled.[2] Acupuncture anesthesia is least satisfactory when used in abdominal surgery because of this traction and also because strong abdominal muscles do not become sufficiently relaxed. In slender patients and under gentle surgical technique, acupuncture is sufficient anesthesia.[3]

One of the adverse effects of acupuncture is its painlessness, which is also one of its most appealing aspects. Even the calming of pain is not

[1] "A Prickly Panacea Called Acupuncture," *Life*, LXXI (August 13, 1972), 35.
[2] *Acupuncture Anaesthesia* (Peking: Foreign Languages Press, 1972), p. 7.
[3] E. Gray Dimond, "Acupuncture Anesthesia," *The Journal of the American Medical Association*, CCXVIII (December 6, 1971), 1561.

a cure, and a poorly diagnosing practitioner can do more harm than good. Furthermore, a practitioner who is ignorant of the power of acupuncture points can jeopardize the health or life of his patient. The points have as much potential for harm as for healing. Dangerous points on a pregnant woman can induce a hemorrhage. Other points are hazardous for asthmatics taking cortisone or for cardiac patients.[4] A recent Russian medical report introduces another adverse possibility: "A Rare Case of Carcinoma of the Skin Arising after Acupuncture (Case Report)."[5]

Still, the most dangerous possibility is the fake or unwise acupuncturist himself. "One misplaced needle can kill in a matter of hours. I have had patients sent to me who were almost dead from other acupuncturists," remarked one practitioner.[6] Many sincere masters of acupuncture fear that inadequate teachers will show the location of a few points to novices excited by the newness of acupuncture. This would lead to unsafe practices, and acupuncture would fall into the hands of quacks.[7] Hence there is a belief among legitimate acupuncturists that a Medical Doctor degree should be required for acupuncture practice, that the Chinese art should be put into Western medical schools. Formerly acupuncture was mostly a family tradi-

[4] Henriette Chandet, "Les Aiguilles Mystérieuses," *Paris Match*, No. 1190 (February 26, 1972), 58–61.

[5] See I. M. Tsukerman, "A Rare Case of Carcinoma of the Skin Arising after Acupuncture (Case Report)," *Voprosy Onkologii*, XVI (1970), 88.

[6] "A Prickly Panacea," *loc. cit.*

[7] Eileen Simpson, "Acupuncture (à la française)," *Saturday Review*, LV (February 19, 1972), 49.

tion passed down through the generations. Today, under typical schoolroom conditions and after intensive training, a knowledge of acupuncture techniques might be achieved within three years.

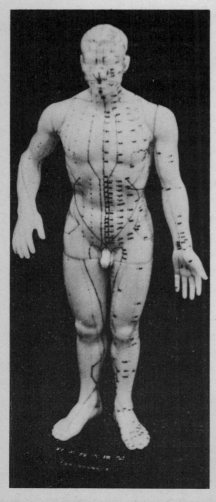

Figure 39. Chinese figurine with acupuncture meridians and points.

A great deal of experience and judgment would be necessary after these three years for true skill in acupuncture.

There are many well-established schools of

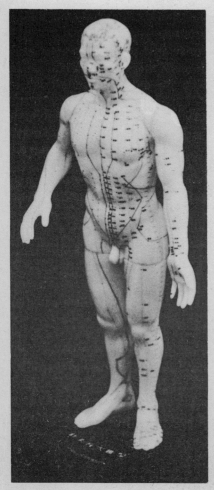

Figure 40.
Chinese
figurine with
acupuncture
meridians
and points.

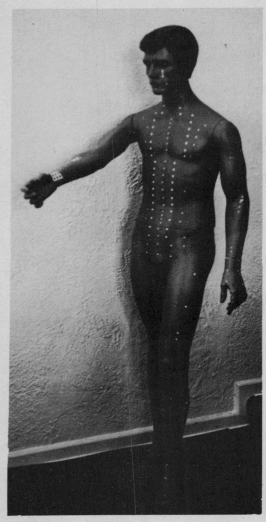

Figure 41. A life-size model with
the acupuncture points.

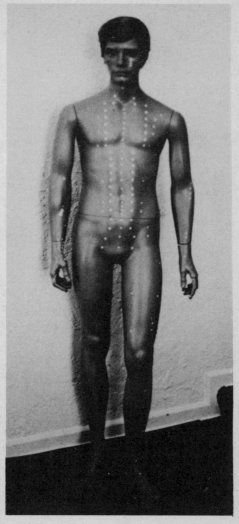

Figure 42. A life-size model with the acupuncture points.

acupuncture throughout the world, mainly in Asia and Europe. These colleges offer three- or four-year courses in acupuncture practice. Both approaches to acupuncture are taught, treatment by formula and treatment by the traditional methods of diagnosis.

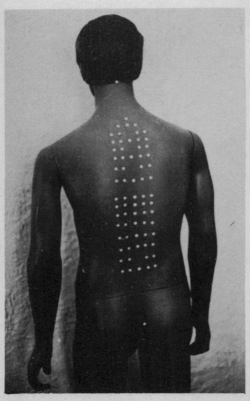

Figure 43. A life-size model with the acupuncture points (back view).

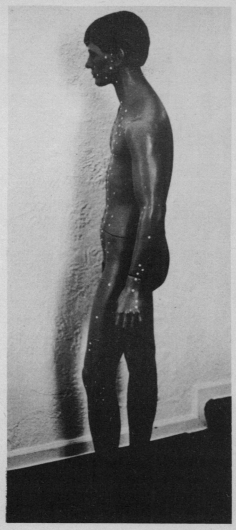

Figure 44. A life-size model with
the acupuncture points
(side view).

CHAPTER TEN

The
Future

Although most fads fade away with the passage of time, acupuncture (for, indeed, it too has become a fad) does not seem likely to follow this trend. Serious medical men have realized the value of an Oriental-Western medical approach. The American Medical Association has already sent invitations to China requesting that Chinese surgeons be sent to the United States in order to attend AMA-sponsored meetings for the demonstration of acupuncture techniques. President Nixon's personal physician, Dr. Walter Robert Tkach, while in Peking asked that groups of American doctors be allowed to have first hand training on acupuncture anesthesia in China.[1] Already operations involving acupuncture anesthesia have taken place successfully in the United States. Several states have legalized the practice of acupuncture done by non-licensed doctors, i.e., by traditional acupuncturists. Research to explain acupuncture is continuing throughout the world, and many questions may be answered in a few years.

[1] "Nixon M.D. Acclaims Acupuncture," *Star-News*, April 12, 1972, p. 5.

The eventual acceptance of acupuncture is inevitable because *acupuncture works*. The quest for health and physical well-being is unending. It has long inspired new attitudes in medicine, and it will inspire Western acceptance of the healing art of acupuncture. Those who seek relief from pain or illness may find their relief through acupuncture treatments. Acupuncture's healing value is not dependent on drugs or substances foreign to the body, but helps the body to rebalance its own energy and hence cure itself. To a world apprehensive of drugs and their toxic side effects, acupuncture provides an alternative, natural healing.

The following case histories are a few examples of the great healing power of acupuncture.

Case History 1

HISTORY

The patient was a man approximately sixty-six years old. He complained of excruciating pain in the left shoulder and the lower back for over three years. The patient's physician had informed him that he was suffering from chronic subdeltoid bursitis in the left shoulder and from the dislocation of an invertebral disk in the back. The patient had been unable to find permanent relief from his pain. (Chronic bursitis is resistant to medical therapy.)

ACUPUNCTURE TREATMENT

The patient was first seen in late 1971. His condition required an increase of Yin force in the body.

Needling of:

Tso-chien-yü 左肩俞 on the large-intestine meridian, a point near the joint of the shoulder blade and the collar bone.

Ch'ü-ch'ih 曲池 on the large-intestine meridian, a point near the elbow on the posterior of the arm.

Yao-yü 腰俞 on the governor-vessel meridian, a point near the base of the spine.

Each treatment lasted from ten to fifteen minutes.

RESULTS

The patient was treated every five days over a period of two weeks. He received a total of three treatments. After this time he was relieved of all former pain. The pains have never since recurred.

Case History 2

HISTORY

The patient was a man approximately fifty years old. He had suffered severe pains, muscle weakness, and limitation of motion in the neck, arms, and back for twenty years. Poor circulation in the arms and muscle spasms were also present. The patient had been informed that he was suffering from chronic bursitis. His doctors had given him various forms of medical treatment, but all therapy was only temporarily effective. The intensity of pain made daily usage of codeine necessary.

ACUPUNCTURE TREATMENT

The patient's personal physician encouraged him to undergo acupuncture treatment since medical therapy was unable to cure him. The patient was first seen in early 1972.

Increase of Yang:

> Needling of *Ta-ch'ui* 大椎 on the governor-vessel meridian, a point on the spine between the two shoulder blades.

Increase of Yin:

Needling of:

> *Tso-chien-yü* 左肩俞 on the large-intestine meridian, a point near the joint of the shoulder blade and the collar bone.

Ch'ü-ch'ih 曲池 on the large-
intestine meridian, a point near the elbow
on the posterior of the arm.

Each treatment lasted from ten to fifteen minutes.

RESULTS

The patient was treated once a week over a
period of two weeks. He received two treatments
and was relieved of all pain. He did not take nor
did he need one pain reliever since then. There
was no further limitation of motion, and the patient
was able to do things which he had formerly been
unable to do because of his disease.

Case History 3

HISTORY

The patient was a fifty-five-year-old woman.
She had undergone a series of upper gastrointestinal X-rays at her community hospital. The radiologist reported that "a definite gastric ulcer was
demonstrated which was quite large." The patient
was then advised by one medical doctor to enter
the hospital for immediate medical treatment.
However, with the approval of her personal physician, she sought acupuncture treatment.

ACUPUNCTURE TREATMENT

The patient was first seen in early 1972.
Both needling and moxibustion were used to increase the Yang force in the body.

Needling of:

Nei-kuan 内関 on the pericardium (vascular system) meridian, a point near the wrist on the anterior of the arm.

Chung-wan 中脘 on the conceptional-vessel meridian, a point on the upper abdomen.

Tzu-san-li 足三里 on the stomach meridian, a point below the knee on the outer side of the leg.

Moxibustion:
Three times at *Yao-yü* 腰俞 on the governor-vessel meridian, a point near the base of the spine.

Each treatment lasted from twenty to thirty minutes.

RESULTS

The patient was treated twice a week over a period of six weeks. She received a total of twelve treatments. After this time she took another series of upper gastrointestinal X-rays. There was no hint of the former huge gastric ulcer. In the words of the radiologist:

If one nitpicks he may conclude that there is some coarsening of the mucosal folds of the previous ulcer, but there is no evidence of residual ulcer and I do not even see any real evidence of residual cicatricial change through this area. Elsewhere, the findings remain normal as previously.

Impression: The patient has had a giant benign gastric ulcer which is healed since the last time we examined her.

Within forty days the ulcer had been completely healed.

Case History 4

HISTORY

The patient was a man of sixty-five. He had suddenly developed a case of tinnitus aurium (a subjective sensation of ringing in the ears). His physician was unable to determine the cause of the tinnitus. The patient underwent various medical treatments and was given tranquilizers. However, these were unable to help him.

ACUPUNCTURE TREATMENT

The patient was first seen within one week after the ringing sensation began. This was in early 1967. His condition required an increase of Yang force in the body.

Needling of:

T'ing-hui 聽 會 on the gallbladder meridian, a point on the side of the face near the ear lobe.

T'ing-kung 聽 宮 on the small-intestine meridian, a point on the side of the face near the tragus of the ear.

I-feng 翳 風 on the triple-heater meridian, a point on the neck behind the ear lobe.

Each treatment lasted from twenty to twenty-five minutes.

RESULTS

The patient was treated twice a week over a period of two weeks. He received a total of three treatments. After this time the ringing in his ears ceased completely and never returned.

Case History 5

HISTORY

The patient was an eight-year-old boy. A few weeks after birth he had undergone operations to correct a harelip. Since that time he had suffered from deafness. A series of eighth-nerve X-rays were taken when the patient was five years old. These showed that the loss of hearing was due to conduction deafness—deafness due to defect of the sound-conducting apparatus: the auditory meatus, the ear drum, or the auditory ossicles. The report of the radiologist was as follows.

There is symmetry of the internal acoustic canals with mild narrowing on the left as compared to the right. There is presence of normal appearing cochlea and vestibular apparatus bilaterally. There is asymmetry in the appearance of the auditory ossicles with suggestion of interruption of the ossicle chain on the right. No erosions in the region of the tympanic antrum are observed.

Conclusion: Asymmetry in appearance of the ossicles, otherwise negative eighth nerve study.

ACUPUNCTURE TREATMENT

The patient was first seen in early 1972. His condition required an increase of Yang force.

Needling of:

T'ing-hui 聽會 on the gall-bladder meridian, a point on the side of the face near the ear lobe.

I-feng 翳風 on the triple-heater meridian, a point on the neck behind the ear lobe.

Each treatment lasted from fifteen to twenty minutes.

RESULTS

The patient was treated twice a week over a period of six weeks. He received a total of twelve treatments. After this time hearing tests were again given by the patient's physician. They demonstrated that the patient's hearing had improved by 25 percent.

Case History 6

HISTORY

The patient was a thirty-year-old man. He had suffered from a skin allergy for twenty years. Itching, redness of the skin, and wheals would develop over his body, especially in the facial area. His physician had diagnosed the ailment as chronic urticaria. Although the patient's diet was restricted, the symptoms of urticaria recurred periodically. No specific cause of the allergy was identified.

ACUPUNCTURE TREATMENT

The patient was seen in late 1971. His condition required an increase of Yang force in the body.

Needling of:

Ch'ü-ch'ih 曲池 on the large-intestine meridian, a point near the elbow on the posterior of the arm.

Feng-shih 風市 on the gall-bladder meridian, a point on the middle of the outer thigh.

The treatment lasted twenty minutes.

RESULTS

The patient was given only one treatment. After this he had no dietetic restrictions and suffered no recurrence of his former symptoms.

Case History 7

HISTORY

The patient was a seventy-year-old woman, with no history of eye diseases. She suddenly developed diplopia (double vision). Her ophthalmologist was unable to help her.

ACUPUNCTURE TREATMENT

The patient was first seen in mid-1972. Her condition required the balancing of Yang and Yin at two points. Equal amounts of stimulation and reduction were given at the two points.

Needling of:

Tsuan-chu 攢竹 on the bladder meridian, a point on the tip of the eye brow above the nose.

Ch'ing-ming 晴明 on the bladder meridian, a point between the bridge of the nose and the lacrimal caruncle.

Each treatment lasted twenty-five minutes.

RESULTS

The patient received a total of two treatments within one week. After this time her vision returned to normal.

Case History 8

HISTORY

The patient was a forty-three-year-old woman. She had suffered from the symptoms of influenza and from coughing for over one and one-half years. Influenza had been complicated by secondary bacterial infection of the lung. The patient's physician suspected that bacterial pneumonia had set in. The patient was taking various antitussive medications.

ACUPUNCTURE TREATMENT

The patient was first seen in late 1971. Her condition required an increase of Yin force in the body.

Needling of:

Ho-ku 合谷 on the large-intestine meridian, a point on the hand in the "web" between the forefinger and the thumb.

Ch'ü-ch'ih 曲池 on the large-intestine meridian, a point near the elbow on the posterior of the arm.

Each treatment lasted twenty minutes.

RESULTS

The patient was treated twice a week over a period of three weeks. She received a total of five treatments. After this time fever, coughing, and other influenza symptoms no longer recurred.

Case History 9

HISTORY

The patient was a forty-five-year-old man. He had suffered from pain and limitation of motion in the neck and shoulders for over one month. A sudden wrench of the neck had precipitated these symptoms. Physicians diagnosed his case as the cervical root compression syndrome; there was a pinched nerve between the fifth and sixth cervical vertebrae. The patient was forced to wear an iron collar in order to maintain continuous immobilization of his neck.

ACUPUNCTURE TREATMENT

The patient was first seen in the summer of 1971. His condition required an increase of Yin force in the body.

Needling of:

Pai-lao 百勞 , an extra point lying beyond the meridians, a point at the base of the hairline on either side of the cervical vertebrae.

Each treatment lasted thirty minutes.

RESULTS

The patient received a total of two treatments over a period of one week. After this time the patient experienced no further pain, stiffness, or limitation of motion in the neck and shoulder areas. He no longer needed the iron collar.

Case History 10

HISTORY

The patient was a fifteen-year-old boy. He had suffered from nocturnal enuresis (bed-wetting) for seven years. Both urologists and psychiatrists had been unable to correct the disorder. The patient had been given a variety of drugs, including tranquilizers and drugs to promote lighter sleep. However, he continued to wet his bed.

ACUPUNCTURE TREATMENT

The patient was first seen in late 1969. His condition required an increase of Yin force in the body.

Needling of:

Kuan-yüan 関元 on the conceptional meridian, a point on the umbilical region of the abdomen.

Shen-yü 腎俞 on the bladder meridian, a point on the back on the waistline.

Each treatment lasted twenty minutes.

RESULTS

The patient received a total of two treatments over a period of one week. After this time the enuresis stopped. The patient and his parents were very grateful, and they were able to develop a better relationship.

Case History 11

HISTORY

The patient was a fifty-five-year-old woman. She had suffered from vaginal leukorrhea (non-bloody vaginal discharge) for approximately six years. After menopause the vaginal tissues are thin and lack normal resistance. Infection by various organisms can cause leukorrhea. The patient's physicians were unable to control the leukorrhea.

ACUPUNCTURE TREATMENT

The patient was first seen in early 1968. Her condition required an increase of Yang force in the body.

Needling of:

Kuan-yüan 関元 on the conceptional meridian, a point on the umbilical region of the abdomen.

Chung-chi   中極   on the conceptional meridian, a point on the umbilical
region of the abdomen below Kuan-yüan.

Each treatment lasted thirty minutes.

RESULTS

The patient received a total of two treatments
over a period of one week. After this time the discharge stopped.

Case History 12

HISTORY

The patient was a sixty-two-year-old woman.
She had suffered from mild heart failure resulting
in high diastolic blood pressure for eight years.
The patient's heart was doing more work to maintain the required output of blood. Her physician
had prescribed medications to decrease sodium and
water retention (diuretics). One of the diuretics
was Aldomet®, an aldosterone inhibitor. However,
the patient complained of dizziness whenever she
took the medications.

ACUPUNCTURE TREATMENT

The patient was first seen in early 1969. Her condition required an increase of Yin force in the body.

Needling of:

Wei-chung 委中 on the bladder meridian, a point on the back of the knee.

Tzu-san-li 足三里 on the stomach meridian, a point below the knee on the outer side of the leg.

Each treatment lasted thirty minutes.

RESULTS

The patient was treated every third day over a period of two weeks. She received a total of five treatments. After this time the diastolic pressure dropped to normal, and other functions of the heart were normal.

Case History 13

HISTORY

The patient was a forty-three-year-old woman. She had suffered from insomnia for three years.

She was not able to fall asleep unless she took four sleeping pills each night. Even then sleep did not come until several hours later. After a fall which she attributed to her drugged condition, the patient stopped taking medication. At this point sleep was virtually impossible. She sought acupuncture treatment immediately.

ACUPUNCTURE TREATMENT

The patient was first seen in mid-1972. Her condition required an increase of Yang force in the body.

Needling of:

Shen-men 神門 on the heart meridian, a point on the wrist on the anterior of the arm.

The treatment lasted twenty minutes.

RESULTS

The patient was given only one treatment. That night, thinking that the acupuncture treatment might not be effective, she took one sleeping pill. She fell asleep within one hour, and her sleep was deep and unbroken. After that time the patient took no further medication and suffered no difficulty in sleeping.

With a record for healing like this, acupuncture cannot be ignored. The world will come to esteem acupuncture as highly as the Chinese have for the last five thousand years. Acupuncture has been practiced not only as a cure for specific diseases but also as a principle for general health. One may sum up the entire philosophy of acupuncture and Chinese healing by recalling the ancient Mandarins, who paid their physicians to keep them in good health. When they fell into illness, they immediately stopped all payment.[2] Acupuncture is, above all, preventive medicine, and the patient is treated as a whole—body, mind, and spirit inseparable. There is a precept which applies to acupuncture as well as to all Chinese healing; the acupuncturist will admonish, "Curing is not so good as preventing, and preventing is not so good as taking care of oneself."

[2] Henriette Chandet, "Les Aiguilles Mystérieuses," *Paris Match*, No. 1190 (February 26, 1972), 58–61.

SUMMARY OF YANG AND YIN

YANG FORCE	YIN FORCE

Qualities

Plus	Minus
Light	Dark
Hot	Cold
Man	Woman
The urge to grow outward	The urge to shrink inward
Sol phase	Gel phase

Organs and Meridians

Stomach	Heart
Large intestine	Liver
Small intestine	Kidneys
Bladder	Spleen (pancreas)
Gallbladder	Lungs
Triple heater (hypothalamus)	Pericardium (vascular system)
Meet at the head running near surface of the skin	Meet at the chest running deeper under the skin

Symptoms

Pain	Paralysis
Burning sensation	Cold
Spasms	Laxity
Overactivity	Underactivity
Excess	Deficiency

YANG FORCE	YIN FORCE

Pulses

Small intestine	Heart
Gallbladder	Liver
Bladder	Kidneys
Large intestine	Lungs
Stomach	Spleen
Triple heater (hypothalamus)	Circulation (pericardium)

GLOSSARY

Acupuncture

針灸

The traditional Chinese art of healing. It involves the insertion of needles into special points on the body (needling), the concentration of pressure at these points (*an na*), and the burning of herbs on or near the body (*moxa*). Acupuncture has also been developed as an effective anesthetic.

Ai

艾

Dried wormwood or *Artemesia,* the herb used in moxibustion.

An Na

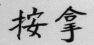

A prolonged concentration of pressure at an acupuncture point. The pressure is caused by the hands or by *an na* instruments. Another aspect of *an na* is the production of an electrical charge on the body which discharges itself at an acupuncture point.

Chen Chiu

針 灸

Chia I Ching

甲乙經

An Introduction to Acupuncture and Moxibustion, written around 250 A.D. This work lists 649 acupuncture points on the body. It was very influential in China and throughout the world as a reference on acupuncture.

Ch'i

氣

A bipolar energy arising from the interaction of Yang and Yin. In the human body, *ch'i* is the vital force and life essence. Any imbalance of *ch'i* causes disease or pain in the body.

Conceptional-Vessel Meridian

任脉

The meridian running up the front center of the body. It exerts influence over all six Yin organ meridians.

Five Elements

五行

According to Taoist philosophy, the fundamental constituents of the universe: wood, fire, earth, metal, water. The five elements are related by complex cycles.

Fen

分

A unit of measurement used in acupuncture, one-tenth of a personal inch or *ts'un*.

Gel Phase

One of the two phases of a colloid (a suspension of minute particles). The *gel* phase represents the tendency of the particles to coalesce and join together.

Governor-
Vessel Meridian

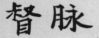

The meridian running up the back center of the body and over the head. It exerts influence over all six Yang organ meridians.

K'o Cycle

A cyclical relation between the five elements. It is a cycle of control or subjugation in which each element subdues the next but one.

Meridian

A path of *ch'i* on the surface level of the body. The acupuncture points lie on the meridians, and the body's *ch'i* is rebalanced by acupuncture treatment at these points. There are fourteen meridians on the body—twelve organ meridians, the conceptional-vessel meridian, and the governor-vessel meridian.

Moxa

艾絨

The burning of herbs on or near the body (moxibustion).

Moxibustion

艾灸

The burning of an herb (*ai*) on or near the body to give strength or to stimulate.

Nei Ching

内經

Book of Internal Medicine, the most ancient medical text of China, written over five thousand years ago. The *Nei Ching* has an entire section on acupuncture points, meridians, needles, and diseases curable by acupuncture.

Pien

砭

A piece of sharp stone. In the premetal era in China, diseases were cured by pricking certain points on the body with the *pien.* This was the early form of acupuncture.

Punctoscope

A machine which registers electrical microcurrents. By utilizing the electrical properties of acupuncture points, the punctoscope can locate the acupuncture points.

Sheng Cycle

生

A cyclical relation between the five elements. It is a cycle of generation, of a "mother-child" relationship. Wood engenders fire; fire engenders earth; earth engenders metal; metal engenders water; water engenders wood.

Sol Phase

One of the two phases of a colloid (a suspension of minute particles). The *sol* phase represents the tendency of the particles to repel each other and spread.

Taking
the Pulse

按脉

A complicated and important part of diagnosis. The skilled acupuncturist is able to ascertain the conditions of the twelve organs, the patient's blood pressure, and the health of the entire organism.

Tao

道

The entirety of active and inactive operations (Yang and Yin) constituting the course of the universe. The philosophy of the ancient Chinese sages, Divine Reason or the path of understanding.

Ts'un

寸

The unit of measurement in acupuncture, a personal inch differing from individual to individual.

Wormwood

The herb which is burned in moxibustion, called *ai* by the Chinese.

Yang

陽

A principle or force representing the urge to grow outward. Also, the positive, the bright, the warm, the male concept.

Yin

陰

A principle or force representing the urge to shrink inward. Also, the negative, the dark, the cool, the female concept. The universe represents the interplay of the two activities, Yang and Yin, and their vicissitudes.

BIBLIOGRAPHY

Anonymous. *Acupuncture Anaesthesia*. Peking: Foreign Languages Press, 1972.

——. "The Chinese Surgeons." *Newsweek*, LXXVII (June 7, 1971), 78.

——. "The Mutes Regain Their Speech." *China Reconstructs*, XXI (February, 1972), 7–10.

——. "Nixon M.D. Acclaims Acupuncture." *Star-News*, April 12, 1972, 5.

——. "A Prickly Panacea Called Acupuncture." *Life*, LXXI (August 13, 1971), 32–35.

——. "Yang, Yin and Needles." *Time*, XCVIII (August 9, 1971), 37–38.

Chandet, Henriette. "Les Aiguilles Mystérieuses." *Paris Match*, Number 1190 (February 26, 1972), 58–61.

Cusack, Michael. "Acupuncture—Is Getting the Needle Good for You?" *Science World*, XXIV (May 15, 1972), 9–13.

Dimond, E. Gray, M.D. "Acupuncture Anesthesia." *The Journal of the American Medical Association*, CCXVIII (December 6, 1971), 1558–1563.

Heroldová, Dana. *Acupuncture and Moxibustion*. New York: Altai Press, 1968.

Lawson-Wood, Denis, and Joyce Lawson-Wood. *The Five Elements of Acupuncture and Chinese Massage*. Russington, Sussex, England: Health Science Press, 1966.

Simpson, Eileen. "Acupuncture (à la française)," *Saturday Review*, LV (February 19, 1972), 47–49.